LIFE IN THE BLOOD

A Story of Miraculous Healing

Devena LaSha Witherspoon

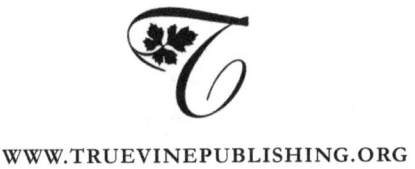

WWW.TRUEVINEPUBLISHING.ORG

Life In The blood
By Devena LaSha Witherspoon

Published by
True Vine Publishing Co.
810 Dominican Dr.
Nashville, TN 37228
www.TrueVinePublishing.org

ISBN: 978-1-962783-69-9 Paperback
ISBN: 978-1-962783-70-5 eBook

Printed in the United States of America—First printing.

TABLE OF CONTENTS

The Lump

I didn't grow up with much, but I grew up with everything that mattered—discipline, faith, and the kind of love that showed up every single day, even when money didn't.

Growing up in Northern Mississippi, I enjoyed sunny summers eating watermelons on the front porch with my six siblings. Spring was the time for family and friends to reunite at the Railroad Festival to eat BBQ and funnel cakes while watching the children scream on the carnival rides. Fall was only for football. Winter was spent looking out the window hoping for snow—even if it were only a few snowflakes.

As seasons and the events aforementioned are somewhat predictable, life is not. Growing up in a large family, life brought about many surprises and unusual circumstances. As a young girl, I did not have my own bed; I shared it with my youngest sister. Most nights, I was fearful that I would force her little body off the bed, so I would sleep very close to the edge of the mattress, thickened by old blankets. We wore clothes given to us by friends in the neighborhood. We dealt with tornadoes, air conditioners in the window, running to the bus stop—and sometimes even walking to school.

But none of this hindered my parents from having all seven of their children in church five days out of the week. My parents were strict but loving. My father was a towering, Goliath-figure in my childhood, even though he only stood 5 foot, 4 inches. He embodied the discipline imparted into him from his military training. My father was a disciplined man, running five miles nearly every day. Daily, he would instill these disciplines in my siblings and me. Being punctual was very important to my father; so, he put rules in place that would help us to be on time. We had to clean the house and iron our clothes at night; and we had to make our beds before leaving for school each morning.

My mother was stern, yet she displayed an angelic presence in our daily lives. She supported our father's military-like regiment, making sure we were always groomed and clean. But Mama was also the fun parent who played with us, making sure that we never lost the joy of childhood. I'll always remember my mother playing basketball in the backyard, shooting three-pointers into the basketball hoop nailed to the light pole.

My parents were devoted Pentecostal preachers. They were sure to have us read the Bible and pray daily.

My mother preached the gospel of Jesus Christ all over Northern Mississippi and Alabama; and for this, she was given the nickname: "The Bootleg Missionary." When she was called into the ministry, she had young children under the age of five. During the early 1980s, a woman with young children was usually not ordained in the Church of God in Christ nor permitted to travel to minister. My parents focused on imparting biblical principles like living a holy life and the power of prayer. To ensure we practiced what was preached, each day after school, my father gave us instructions to meet in my brothers' bedroom to pray in tongues for 30 minutes.

"Repeat after me," my father would say in his military tone, "shin-shin shun-do hya-b-hya."

In unison, seven little voices would cry out, "shin-shin shun-do hya-b-hya."

We were too young to understand what we were doing, but we dare not question commands given to us by our father. As we said this phrase over and over, my siblings and I looked at each other, confused, with smirk grins on our greasy faces. After speaking in tongues for several minutes, we would begin to sing 'shin-shin shun-do hya-b-hya' in the key of A-flat. At first, we would begin singing the same notes and then eventually sing in three-part harmony—all a cappella. After 10 minutes, my father would usually leave the double-wide trailer to purchase a Coca-Cola before dinner.

When it seemed safe, one of the younger siblings would yell, "He Comin-in-a-honda!!"

Not having a mature understanding of the powerful gift of speaking in tongues, we would laugh hysterically. If my mother heard us laughing, we would hear her heavy footsteps marching across the living room.

"I don't hear y'all praying," Mom would yell as she made her way from the kitchen towards the bedroom. Immediately we would begin to scream loudly, "shin-shin shun-do hya-b-hya."

Upon completing our 30 minutes of prayer, we all would have to sign a form stating the start time and finish time of praying. After prayer and homework, all seven of us would eat together at the dining room table each night. At this oval table, we discussed what the teachers taught during class, band rehearsals, after-school sports, any material that needed to be purchased for a special school project and even compared lunch food in the cafeteria to the food Mama Linda prepared for us. We were taught to look out for one another and to always tell the truth. When one child got into trouble, we all were disciplined… and there was no such thing as 'time-out.'

Our parents commanded that if we left the house with someone, we were to return home with that same person. We were not allowed to participate in sleepovers or anything that our parents deemed ungodly. My mother drilled the importance of treating each other with respect and always to love the Lord. These core values played an important role in my life when I was diagnosed with stage 3 Non-Hodgkin's Lymphoma in June 2017.

I'll never forget that sunny Saturday evening when I arrived at home with my best friend. Earlier that day, we had brunch at a nice, quiet restaurant in a nearby city. We laughed and talked for hours and only requested coffee refills until the restaurant stopped serving food. Once arriving at my home and sitting on the couch, we continued our conversation for several hours without missing a beat. Because we had not seen each other in several years, we had so much to catch up on. Before she left, she prayed for me, my husband, and blessed our home. Her hug was so warm and electrifying it brought me to tears.

As I closed the door behind her, I began to sing praise to God all over my house. I walked upstairs to my bathroom to begin doing my hair and noticed a large knot had appeared on my chest. The oval, pear-like lump had appeared under my right collarbone without warning. It was not there when I woke up that morning and I had not felt anything throughout the day. I knew immediately that something was wrong and Facetimed my mother.

As always, I screamed, "Hey, Sis Gilleylen!"

"Hey, daughter! WHAT'S THAT?????" Mama yelled!

The lump was so large it could be seen through the phone. I explained to my mother that I didn't know what this large mass was and that it had just appeared out of nowhere.

"Does it hurt?" Mom asked.

I pressed on it and softly said, "No."

With all the authority she could muster up, even through her tears, she began to pray for me. She called on the name of Jesus with so much compassion and courage. Her words of healing pierced my heart because I could feel her talking to God face-to-face on my behalf.

"You go to the doctor Monday morning to see what's going on with you!" she commanded with her lips pressed tightly together.

Being the obedient child that I am, I did exactly what she said. I went to the doctor, who performed a series of X-rays and other examinations. My husband and I waited anxiously in the cold, sterile waiting room for the doctor to come back with the results.

The doctor's face was pale and warped with concern. My heart began to pound—he clearly did not have good news.

"Mr. and Mrs. Witherspoon, I'm sorry, there are no private rooms. We can go into this stockroom if you don't mind discussing your results."

The doctor walked us into the tight stockroom filled with boxes of medical supplies.

"I'm Dr. Evans. The results from your X-rays have come in, and from what I see, I would strongly suggest that you see an oncologist."

"What is an oncologist?" I asked, with a look of absolute confusion.

He looked at me as confused as I was looking at him. With a very gentle voice, he said, "An oncologist is a cancer doctor."

I went into shock. I looked at my husband, and he looked shocked as well. I smiled at the doctor and told him that I felt fine and was not in any pain. In my mind, he was clearly mistaken. There was no way I had cancer.

Dr. Evans offered a sympathetic smile. "I'll have the nurse call you with my referral."

Dr. Evans was not a specialist in cancer, so he could not offer any advice or counsel—only a referral.

The oncologist meeting was set a month away. The next 30 days were filled with research and exercise. After discovering a family history of cancer in my grandfather and aunts on both sides, I was determined. I would break the chain of this generational curse. I fervently prayed and fasted, giving no room for negative thoughts. I would never even speak the word "cancer" out of my mouth. I only researched healthy holistic living and never the symptoms nor results of cancer. I was going to beat this cancer before I ever met the oncologist.

The day I met the oncologist, I was nervous; my hands were sweaty, and my legs were shaking uncontrollably. My husband, Thaddeus, and I were led to the oncologist's office by the receptionist. The numerous degrees, awards, and certifications that filled the wall didn't settle my queasy stomach. As he introduced himself to me, I noticed from his dialect that he was from another country.

"Where are you from?" I asked to break the tension in the room.

"I'm from Germany," the doctor said proudly.
I enthusiastically shared with the doctor that my dad was in the military, and I was born in Germany. We talked for what seemed like 45 minutes. We discussed family history, church, and my daily routine. I also said that I was not in pain, nor did I feel tired.

"Are you losing weight?" the white-haired doctor asked.

I gladly shouted, "YES!"

His next question scared me a little bit. "Are you losing weight with little to no effort?"

I sat straight up in my chair and, with trembling in my voice, I said, "Yes. Is that a good thing?"

"No. We must do a biopsy to determine what this protruding mass is," he said with a look of devastation.

The oncologist instructed the nurse to schedule me as soon as possible for a biopsy. I was so disappointed that I was in the hospital having this procedure. I was a healthy person, so in my mind, I only planned to be in the hospital to have a baby. I never imagined my first hospital visit would be like this.

Once I was prepped for the procedure, I was rolled back to a sterile room. It was so cold, and every medical instrument was squeaky clean. The room resembled the hospital shows I used to watch on television. I was transferred to another, less comfortable and cold bed. A new doctor introduced himself to me and described what he was about to do. All was going well until he lifted the foot-long needle off the table.

"Are you going to use that?" I screamed. "Somebody go get my mama!" I yelled hysterically.

"Don't worry. We're going to use some numbing medicine. It won't be as bad as it looks," he said with a smile.

He smeared some cold, brown odorless liquid onto the large mass on my chest. Then one of the assistants handed him that long needle.

"You're gonna feel a pinch, then some pressure. Hold still and breathe out," the doctor whispered.

He placed the needle on my chest and pressed downward. I felt the sting of the needle, but more of the pressure he used to push through the mass. He pulled a sample of tissue through the needle and placed it on the tray next to me.

"We're all done," he said with a smile on his face. "We should have the results in a couple of days."

I returned to the oncologist two days later for the results. Thaddeus and I waited with anticipation. I mustered all of the faith and belief I had learned from my Pentecostal upbringing, repeating scriptures of healing under my breath.

"By His stripes I am healed."

"I am more than a conqueror."

"He sent His Word and healed me."

"Your faith has made you whole."

Thaddeus lovingly held my hand firmly, quietly girding me with his faith. The wait for the doctor was only five minutes, but it felt like an eternity. My heart jumped when the creaking door slowly opened. I studied the doctor from head to toe, hoping to see some sign of positive news. But I didn't see any.

"Hello, Mr. and Mrs. Witherspoon. I have the results of your biopsy," he said, bypassing any small talk or cordialities.

I braced myself for the news, as it was clear he wasn't bursting with good tidings.

"Unfortunately, we did find cancer. The results of the biopsy revealed that you have stage 3 non-Hodgkin's Lymphoma. It is critical that we start treatment immediately."

I was dumbfounded. I'm usually a thorough person, but I had no questions. All logic and mental processing were absent. Instead, shame began to fill me like the punctured hull of The Titanic. I was raised to believe that faith would overcome any challenge, but my faith did not protect me from cancer. It was like my total walk of faith and salvation was a sham.

Where did I go wrong? I thought.

My mind went back to the days in my brother's room, laughing as we yelled "shin-shin shun-do hya-b-hya." Why didn't all my years of praying in tongues and speaking words of faith work? Why didn't my commitment to singing in the choir and leading praise and worship cause this disease to pass over me? Why me? I was an obedient child, following Ephesians 6:1-2: "Children, obey your parents in the Lord: for this is right. Honour thy father and mother, which is the first commandment with promise."

Who was to blame? I found only one culprit, and it was me. How could I tell my faith-filled mother and father that I was diagnosed with cancer?

After shedding tears and losing my breath, I facetimed my mother.

"Hey Mom," I said, trying to smile.

"What did the doctors say?" my mother questioned.

My mother skipped over our usual shenanigans and went straight for the hardest question she'd ever asked me in the last 37 years.

"Mom, the doctors said it's cancer," I murmured.

"Well, we know God is a healer. We just saw how God healed your brother Cervanties from a stroke five months ago, and He will do the same for you. Stay encouraged and keep me posted on your next visit."

In the following chapters, I'll share the journey of my life—its highs and lows, the struggles I faced, and the victories I achieved. Through each challenge and every moment of growth, I moved closer to healing. Join me as I recount the path that led to personal transformation and peace.

I'm Not Dying

"I'm not dying!" I loudly declared out of the blue with enthusiasm and 100% certainty. Thaddeus' eyes widened with surprise and concern. He rushed to console me.

"No. Of course not! Honey, we will get through this and you're going to come out stronger." He gracefully made this remark while pulling me into his arms, holding me tight. "In fact, we shouldn't even be thinking about death. Let's talk about life. How many kids do we want, and how are we going to build our real estate empire?" His words about our future brought joy and excitement to my heart. The numbness, shame, and disappointment began to melt away like a glacier on a sunny day. My heated determination to live grew stronger, and my desire to live a utopian life with Thaddeus brought tears to my eyes. We laughed and mused about our future from that moment onward.

During the first few months of this journey, I began to appreciate life even more. My passion for life was driven by the words engrafted in my purple Bible. The wrinkled pages, smeared with neon yellow and pink highlighted verses, read: "I shall not die, but live, and declare the works of the Lord." (Psalm 118:17, KJV). I craved to live life to the fullest, and my desire to be whole and healthy grew stronger than before I was diagnosed with cancer. Being placed into the category of a terminally ill patient could not be compared to the awards I obtained in Middle School. I was elected among my peers as 'Most Likely to Succeed' and received a perfect attendance award, just to name a few.

Being in a large family, we were rarely individually recognized because we had to do things together all the time. I felt happy to see the smile on my mother's face in the audience as she gazed at me walking across the stage to receive band awards. But the level of embarrassment after her screaming, "That's my baby!" made my knees shake and terrified the other parents sitting next to her. That degree of shame disappeared as my mother handed me a silver trumpet as her gift to me for being promoted to High School.

My mother was always attentive to our dreams. So, when I shared with her that I dreamed of walking down the main street of Amory, MS, in a denim skirt and a silver trumpet, she made sure that dream came to life.

Receiving those awards and scholarships in Middle School did not seem to have any weight against two words stamped across the top of my medical records: Terminally Ill. But I was reminded of the scripture that "death and life are in the power of the tongue" (Proverbs 18:21, KJV); therefore, I began to speak Faith Confessions daily. Speaking the Word of God regularly catapulted my faith to talk directly to the area that was affected by cancer: my spleen.

According to the Anatomy and Physiology textbook used at Oregon State University, blood transports oxygen and nutrients to the lungs and tissues; forms blood clots to prevent excess blood loss and also carries cells and antibodies that fight infection. This red liquid circulates in the arteries and veins of humans and other vertebrate animals, carrying oxygen to, and carbon dioxide from, the tissues of the body. Red blood cells (erythrocytes) carry oxygen from the lungs to the rest of the body, and white blood cells (leukocytes) help fight infections and aid in the immune process.

The spleen plays a vital role in the immune system, which helps fight against infection. This major organ filters blood where healthy blood cells pass through and circulate through the bloodstream and detects faulty red blood cells causing bacteria or viruses. My scans after chemo and radiation revealed that this organ was almost covered with cancer, so I began to Google 'life without a spleen.' This unofficial research disclosed that I could live a normal life if I chose to have my spleen removed. The radiation oncologist scheduled a consultation with a surgeon on the hospital floor above his office. My mother and I arrived at the hospital on a sunny afternoon and waited patiently in the lobby of the second floor of Vanderbilt Medical Center.

I was very nervous about having surgery. My hands were sweating, and my knees were shaking. The thought of giving someone absolute control of my body to put me to sleep made me nauseous. The thought of leaving the hospital even crossed my mind. I loved to be in control of my life; I guess that's why I never learned how to swim, because relying on the water currents to guide me down the river was not an option; and additionally, I had no faith in a life jacket or the lifeguard.

I have many friends who are nurses, but one of my friends had a husband who is an anesthesiologist. She called me one day and gave me words of wisdom.

'Hey, Sister Witherspoon,' she said in her sweet, professional voice.

'Hello, Evangelist Carswell,' I repeated in the same professional tone.

We both giggled and took a few moments to catch up with each other since I had missed several weeks of church services. Dr. Carswell was recently married, so we giggled about her new life as a wife. We talked about the Lord and how He was sustaining me through this journey.

"Devena," she said with the compassion of a COGIC church mother, "just as you are anointed to sing and work in accounting, we are anointed in the medical field. God has given us a gift, and we use it for His glory. We went to college for medicine, and you attended college for accounting. God has no respect of persons; we just use our gifts in different industries."

And there it was. Peace. I needed this level of tranquility to dismantle the voices in my head and the fear in my heart. It was at this moment I became confident in the prayer my mother prays when she or any of our family members goes to the doctor: "Lord, give the doctors how and what to do. In Jesus' Name, Amen!"

I have no doubt that speaking healing scriptures over my life daily allows me to live a normal life. And with my spleen removed, I will live a healthy life. Oftentimes, we do not use our mouths as instruments given to us for our advantage. Our mouths initiate the sound that our bodies need to hear to come into alignment with the word of God. Elohim—the Creator of the universe—formed our bodies to heal themselves when injured. The doctor assured me that when my spleen was removed, other parts of my body would begin to adjust for my spleen's absence and other organs would begin to filter the blood. God's infinite wisdom begins by His spoken word: 'Let there be...' (Genesis 1:3). Daily, I would declare:

"Body, produce pure blood."

"Red and white blood cells, normalize in Jesus' Name!"

"Nauseousness, go now, in the name of the Lord Jesus Christ!"

"Devil, I dismantle your plot to kill me, to steal from me, and to destroy me. Your weapons and tactics are obliterated in Jesus' Name!"

Romans 10:17 states, "So then faith cometh by hearing, and hearing by the word of God." As I would speak to my body, it was as if a war would begin in my blood. This inward torture escalated to the point I had to go to the ER. My blood pressure registered so high that the doctor refused to let me go home and admitted me into ICU. When I walked into the secluded room, the nurses looked at me with amazement. I could read their thoughts as they looked at my medical charts and then looked back at my brown eyes: "How is she walking in this room instead of being rolled in a wheelchair?" I puzzled the doctor with stroke-level pressure but feeling good.

FAITH CONFESSION:

I command my bones to produce perfect marrow
and my marrow to generate pure Blood!

The Reconciler

Growing up on a bustling street in Amory, Mississippi, I was captivated by the world of criminal law, dreaming of one day becoming a lawyer. In the rare moments when our black-and-white television was available, I would watch *Matlock and Perry Mason*, both of which sparked a deep fascination with legal dramas. These shows ignited my passion for criminal justice, motivating me to attend college in Oxford, MS, where I would pursue a degree in Criminal Justice. My love for proving a point through strong, irrefutable evidence only deepened during those years.

As I matured, I found myself drawn to *Law & Order*, with each episode offering a fresh, intricate case. The unique theme sound, special guest stars, and ever-evolving storylines kept me glued to the screen. The thrill of watching lawyers work tirelessly to win cases against those who broke the law became an obsession. I was driven by the desire to seek justice and punish wrongdoers.

However, my dream of practicing law took an unexpected turn during my senior year of high school. One accounting class changed everything. Throughout school, math had always been my favorite subject, so when I encountered this class, I felt like I had stumbled upon the perfect fusion of numbers and law. The basic concepts of accounting, where income and expense items are allocated into accounts and balanced, felt like the perfect marriage between mathematics and the rules that govern our financial world.

What fascinated me most was the concept of reconciliation. Just like in legal cases, discrepancies in accounting need to be addressed—outstanding items must be reconciled, either by adjusting account balances or deferring certain items to future periods. The meticulous nature of reconciling financial records mirrored the precision I admired in law, and I realized that this world of numbers and order was where I wanted to make my mark.

The scripture that resonates with this process of healing and reconciliation is Romans 5:10: "For if, when we were enemies, we were reconciled to God by the death of His Son, much more, being reconciled, we shall be saved by His life." Through the sacrifice of Jesus on the cross, we are not only reconciled to God but also offered the healing of our bodies. His blood covers our sins and paves the way for us to draw near to God, removing the sting of death as we accept Him as Lord and Savior. This reconciliation brings both spiritual and physical restoration. My own experience of being healed from stage three cancer is a testimony to the power of this truth—by accepting Jesus as my Savior, I received both spiritual peace and physical healing.

Embracing Jesus as my redemptive Savior nullifies the enemy's attempts to claim my soul and unites me with God the Father. Through the reconciliation afforded by His precious blood, I am empowered to overcome fear and operate in the divine authority granted to me through the sacrificial death of Christ on the cross.

Being reconciled by the blood of Jesus opens the door to profound spiritual and practical transformation in our lives. The act of daily confessing Scripture isn't just a ritual—it's a dynamic means of aligning our hearts and minds with God's truth. As we speak His Word, we invite its power into our lives, and in doing so, we begin to manifest the promises He has made to us. His Word becomes more than just text; it becomes a living, powerful force that shapes our thoughts, attitudes, and actions.

The blood of Jesus is the pivotal element in this process of reconciliation, as it bridges the gap between humanity and God, bringing us into right standing with Him. This alignment with God allows us to receive His promises—promises of peace, healing, provision, victory, and eternal life. Through His blood, we are made whole, and our relationship with the Father is restored to what He originally intended. Blood not only cleanses us from sin but also empowers us to live according to His will and to experience the abundant life He has prepared for us.

As we are reconciled through Christ's sacrifice, we are no longer defined by our past mistakes, our fears, or our circumstances. Instead, we are positioned to walk in the fullness of God's blessings. We can claim what the Scripture says we should have—victory over the enemy, divine health, prosperity, joy, and a deep, unshakeable peace. Moreover, the authority we now possess in Christ enables us to live out the calling He has placed on our lives, to act in His power, and to fulfill His purpose for us on this earth. Through the blood of Jesus, we are not only reconciled but empowered to walk in the divine destiny He has ordained for us.

The peace I've found in my faith in God is a profound and unshakable peace that transcends all understanding. It stems from the deep assurance that my mistakes, no matter how grave or numerous, no longer separate me from God's boundless love. His grace, demonstrated through the sacrifice of His only Son, is the bridge that spans the chasm between my imperfections and His perfect holiness. Jesus' atoning death on the cross secured for me not just forgiveness, but access to God's eternal love and mercy, no matter what I've done or where I've been.

Knowing that God, in His infinite love, sent Jesus to rescue me from the destructive schemes of the enemy gives me a peace that is rooted in certainty. Satan's attempts to entrap me in guilt, shame, and fear no longer hold power over me. Through Christ, I have a way out of the snares that would otherwise lead to spiritual and emotional ruin. Jesus is the escape route from the pits of this world—the very pits that were designed by the enemy to rob me of my purpose and to keep me from fulfilling God's plan for my life.

This peace deepens as I set my affections on heavenly

things, as Colossians 3:2 instructs. By fixing my heart on eternal truths rather than fleeting circumstances, I elevate my perspective beyond the temporary struggles of this world. The more I center my thoughts and desires on God's will and His Kingdom, the more I align myself with His purpose for me. This shift in focus propels me to a higher dimension of faith, one that ignites an unrelenting pursuit of God's promises. I begin to see beyond the physical and temporal, and I find myself driven by a deeper conviction to fulfill my calling, knowing that nothing in this world can separate me from the love and purpose God has for me.

As I grow in this peace, I also grow in my resilience. Challenges that once seemed insurmountable now appear as opportunities for God's power to be displayed. I know that no matter the circumstances, I am anchored in a peace that remains constant. This peace allows me to press forward, unwavering and relentless in my pursuit of God's will for my life. It's a peace that empowers me to face life's battles with the confidence that, in Christ, I am already victorious and reconciled.

FAITH CONFESSION:

I am reconciled to The Father through the Blood
of Jesus Christ.

IV

I Am a Mother; Not Barren

All my life, I've dreamed of becoming a mother, longing to hear the sweet words "mom" or "mama" from my own children. As the second oldest in a bustling family of seven, I naturally fell into the role of caregiver. Being the oldest daughter, I was expected to set an example for my younger siblings. It's amusing now, remembering how my eldest brother calls me "big sister," even though I often took charge. My siblings used to call me bossy, but I didn't mind. I was determined to follow my parents' instructions to avoid punishment and maintain order.

This sense of responsibility fueled my desire to marry and become a mother after two years of wedded bliss. My husband, the cherished only child of his mother, was raised to be an exceptional man. I yearned to give him a son, but that dream was cruelly disrupted by an oncologist's diagnosis.

One fateful day, after being admitted to the Intensive Care Unit with stroke-level blood pressure, I was visited by the head of the Oncology department. This doctor, whom I had seen multiple times but always resisted her recommended chemotherapy, approached me differently this time. She arrived on the fourth floor with six students in tow, ready to deliver the grim news from my latest tests. Standing there in her long white coat, she said, "Mrs. Witherspoon, if you don't do something, you're going to die." Her preferred treatment involved a potent dose of chemotherapy. As I listened intently, my mind raced for an escape route.

Then she uttered the words that shattered my heart: "You may want to freeze your eggs."

How could she suggest such a thing? My heart plummeted to my stomach, and a wave of shame washed over me. At 38, childless after 14 years of marriage to my best friend, I felt like an utter failure. The dream of motherhood that I had cherished for so long now seemed to slip through my fingers like sand. I was devastated, my spirit crushed under the weight of disappointment and despair. My faith, once a rock-solid foundation, now felt fragile and uncertain, quivering under the relentless assault of doubt and fear.

We were already financially drained from paying for out-of-pocket holistic treatments, desperately clinging to any hope of a natural miracle. The cost of freezing my eggs would be an insurmountable obstacle. The doctor's words echoed in my mind, amplifying my feelings of inadequacy and helplessness. I couldn't bear the thought of not being able to give my husband the child we both longed for. The shame of failing him, of not fulfilling the role of a mother, gnawed at my soul.

As the doctor's words swirled around in my mind like a

hurricane, I felt the darkness closing in. My faith, which had always been my anchor, was shaken to its core. I questioned everything I had believed in, grappling with the painful reality that my deepest desires might never be realized. My heart was broken, my spirit weary, and my soul cried out for divine intervention in the face of this seemingly insurmountable trial.

Thankfully, I wasn't alone in bearing this devastating news. My dad sat beside me in a recliner while my husband lay on the couch near the restroom. Despite the cartoons playing on the TV, an eerie silence filled the room after the doctor and her students left.

The phrase "freeze your eggs" replayed in my mind like a broken record throughout the night. The next morning, I was discharged from the hospital, but the doctor's words left me entangled in disbelief. Climbing the stairs to our two-story condo, I collapsed onto the bed in a fetal position, silently crying out, "Lord, help me!" Psalm 61:2 echoed in my mind: "When my heart is overwhelmed, lead me to the rock that is higher than I." Unable to speak due to the ache in my heart, I sought solace in scripture.

I found comfort in Psalm 113:9: "He maketh the barren woman to keep house, and to be a joyful mother of children. Praise ye the Lord." I began reciting this verse daily, its words battling the doctor's ominous prediction of early menopause post-chemotherapy.

Watching my mother raise seven children and seeing my siblings with their 18 children deepened my longing for a family. Whenever I babysit my nieces, nephews, and friends' children, I treat them as my own. My love for children grows each time I see their little faces, and with every passing moment, my faith remains steadfast. I trust that one day, my husband and I will conceive. Though it's been 20 years of marriage, God has never failed me.

FAITH CONFESSION:

I am a joyful mother of normal healthy children.

V

I Will Never Lack

Since I was 15, I've been part of the workforce, carving out my own path from a young age. My very first job was as a carhop at Sonic Drive-In, a role I embraced with enthusiasm. There was something deeply rewarding about earning my own money and watching my bank account grow. It wasn't just about the cash—it was about the independence it represented.

My mother played a crucial role in shaping this self-reliance. She raised me to be fiercely independent, teaching me from a young age that while it was important to be self-sufficient, our ultimate dependence should always be on God. She instilled in me a strong work ethic and a belief that I could achieve anything through hard work and faith. Her lessons were simple yet profound: rely on yourself for the day-to-day, but trust in God for guidance and strength.

After graduating from Mississippi State University, I continued to forge my own way, working for three different companies over 25 years. My dedication was unwavering. If I found an employer who shared my values and whom I respected, I stayed loyal and invested in the job. This commitment wasn't just about financial stability—it was a reflection of the independence my mother nurtured in me.

Her influence made me value not only my professional growth but also my personal integrity. I was driven by the desire to prove that I could stand on my own two feet, with the reassurance that my faith would always be my foundation.

Before my diagnosis of stage three lymphoma, I was the epitome of reliability and independence. The pride I felt in my flawless attendance was palpable, like a badge of honor that gleamed brightly against the backdrop of my professional life. I rarely missed work, only taking time off during my paid vacations, and my perfect attendance record mirrored the dedication I had shown throughout high school.

I reveled in the simple joys of robust health, using my insurance only for dental and vision check-ups. My insurance, like a safety net that rarely needed to be deployed, reflected the vitality and well-being I enjoyed. Each visit to the dentist or eye doctor was a reminder of how blessed I was to have my health. The YMCA membership, a benefit from my employer, was more than just a gym membership; it was a sanctuary where I could invigorate my body and mind, enjoying the energizing hum of treadmills and the soothing calm of the pool. In those times of health and security, I took immense pride in my independence. I was deeply proud of my ability to stand on my own and manage my life with such consistency and grace.

This illness struck like a thunderbolt, shattering the very foundation of my life. It didn't just attack my health—it rattled every corner of my existence, from my hard-earned sense of control and independence to the financial security I once took for granted. The need for holistic treatments, crucial for my well-being, exposed a harsh reality: my medical insurance wouldn't cover these costs. I was forced to dig into my own pockets, watching in dismay as my savings dwindled faster than I could keep track.

Desperation gripped me as I turned to the Lord, asking, "Who will take care of me?" The question echoed with a piercing clarity I had never felt before. Financial scarcity was a foreign concept to me; I had always been able to indulge my desires and manage my needs with ease. Money had never been a problem in my adult life. As an accountant, I meticulously managed my company's budget, yet my personal finances were more of a routine than a focus. I contributed steadily to my 401(k) and savings account each month, but when chemotherapy began, my ability to work—and thus my financial stability—came to a halt.

With my insurance plan, there was a three-month waiting period before I could receive any type of disability payment. This monthly disbursement was 40% lower than my regular salary, and all of a sudden, my contribution to my household income was drastically decreased. I did not know of a way to replace that lost income in my current medical condition. Not being able to pay my bills was a deeply embarrassing and humbling experience. The weight of financial strain bore heavily on my shoulders, and putting that type of pressure on my husband, especially within such a short period, was nerve-wracking. The anxiety and fear of not knowing how we would make ends meet kept us up at night.

In those dark and uncertain times, we found our miracle in the word of God. Through prayer and unwavering faith, we discovered a sense of hope and strength that we never knew we had. The scriptures became our beacon of light, guiding us through the storm. Every verse we read, every prayer we uttered, brought us closer together and renewed our spirit. It was through this divine intervention that we found the courage to face our challenges head-on and the reassurance that we were not alone.

As a tither, I always turn to the word of God if my finances are threatened. With boldness, I would declare the words recorded in Psalm 23 and Philippians 4:9 over my money. While alone in my house, I would shout, "God, You will take care of me and supply all of my needs; so I will not lack." As I waited for my next paycheck, I had to completely trust in God to deliver a way of escape.

I recall a vivid moment during the agonizing three-month waiting period when I was visiting my brother in Minneapolis. The morning sun filtered through the curtains, casting a gentle glow on the room as I prepared to head downstairs for breakfast. But first, I decided to take a moment to pray. Kneeling beside the bed, I bowed my head and began to speak to God.

Before I could even finish my first sentence, my cell phone buzzed with a notification. Curious and slightly distracted, I decided to check it. As I swiped past the homepage, a message from Cash App caught my eye. My heart skipped a beat as I opened it and saw that my baby brother had sent me enough funds to cover my mortgage expense.

The relief and gratitude that washed over me were overwhelming. Tears streamed down my face as I began to praise God, my voice cracking with emotion. I cried like a baby, witnessing firsthand the miracle I had prayed for. The room seemed to fill with a warm, comforting presence, and in that moment, I knew we were going to be alright.

For nine long months, I went without a salary from my employer, yet my faith in God's promise from Philippians 4:19 sustained me: "And my God will meet all your needs according to the riches of His glory in Christ Jesus." True to His word, I received unexpected financial support from family and friends. During this challenging period, I was blessed with an international trip to Italy, a gift that brought a much-needed change of scenery. After enduring six grueling months of chemotherapy, my siblings surprised me with a trip to Hawaii. This incredible vacation offered a welcome escape from the monotony of hospital visits and doctor's appointments.

One unforgettable evening in Hawaii, I visited a pineapple plantation. The gentle rumble of the train as it wound through the lush property revealed a breathtaking array of fruits and plants. This peaceful journey through nature's bounty was a poignant reminder of life's beauty and resilience. Later, while sitting on the golden sands of a Hawaiian beach, I felt the warmth of the sun on my skin, mingling with the gentle breeze that carried the salty scent of the sea. The rhythmic lull of the waves rolling in and out created a soothing melody, and the distant cries of seabirds punctuated the tranquil scene. Before me stretched an endless expanse of azure water, sparkling under the bright, clear sky. The horizon was a delicate line where the sea kissed the sky, blending into a soft gradient of blues and greens.

As I sank into the comfort of my beach chair, the tension of recent months seemed to dissolve with each ebbing wave. Despite the storm of lymphoma and the financial strain that had clouded my life, here, in this serene paradise, I found a rare moment of peace. I closed my eyes and let the gentle sound of the ocean wash over me, feeling the soft, warm sand beneath my feet. In this tranquil moment, surrounded by the beauty of nature, I began to reflect on my journey. The words of Psalm 23:2, "He makes me lie down in green pastures; He leads me beside still waters," resonated deeply within me. Here, amidst the stunning landscape, I was experiencing those very "still waters." The peace and calm of this place mirrored the reassurance and comfort I had been seeking during my hardships.

It struck me that, even though my life had been turned upside down, God had provided moments of calm and beauty amidst the chaos. This beach, with its serene waters and sunlit sands, was a living embodiment of the verse that had been a source of solace and strength. It was a reminder that even in the midst of difficulty, I was not abandoned; instead, I was being gently led to places of rest and renewal.

A month after my doctor cleared me to return to work, I was fortunate enough to visit Italy, another beautiful testament to God's provision. My financial needs were met, and I was given the opportunity to explore and appreciate some of the world's most breathtaking places. From the tranquil beaches of Hawaii to the historic splendor of Italy, it was clear that God had not only covered my immediate needs but also allowed me to revel in His magnificent creations. Reflecting on these experiences, I realized that through every trial and triumph, one truth stood unwavering: I will never lack. The divine abundance that had carried me through my darkest times would continue to sustain me, filling my life with grace and wonder.

FAITH CONFESSION:

I do not lack any good thing, for I have more than enough.

VI

I Am Joyful, Not Depressed

Being part of a large family has always been a mixed blessing. As the second of seven children, I often found myself in a position of authority. My older brother and I shared the responsibility of keeping the younger ones in line whenever our parents weren't home. Some called me bossy, but that didn't mean I always got my way. Our household operated like a finely tuned orchestra, each of us with our roles and rhythms. Sharing was not just a practice but a necessity—my four brothers crammed into one room, while my two sisters and I shared another.

Our home was modest but full of life. The creak of the wooden floorboards seemed to narrate the hustle and bustle of seven children preparing for the day. Our bedrooms, though crowded, were decorated with mismatched quilts and family-made crafts. The smell of Mom's cooking—fried potatoes or homemade biscuits—often drifted through the cracked door of our tiny kitchen. The bathroom, however, was a battleground. The walls were painted a pale yellow, chipped in places from years of wear, and a thin shower curtain swayed limply on its rod. The 8x10 mirror above the sink seemed laughably inadequate for three girls trying to style their hair simultaneously. Behind the single door, arguments erupted as we vied for space, while the faint pounding of our brothers' fists added urgency to our morning chaos.

Despite the lack of material wealth, we were rich in love. My parents' daily lessons in biblical principles and their visible displays of affection provided a foundation of security and warmth. **The anxiety of missing holidays with family.**

When I was diagnosed and quarantined, that foundation was shaken. Not being able to host family gatherings or attend our cherished Sunday dinners was one of the most difficult adjustments. I had grown accustomed to the joy and energy of being surrounded by loved ones, and the silence was deafening. My days stretched endlessly, as I battled severe fatigue and loneliness while my husband was at work. Without a job or a hobby to occupy my time, I found myself drawn to the television. I binged crime dramas and thrillers, letting their dark storylines infiltrate my mind. Slowly, I realized I was allowing negativity to take root in my spirit, opening a door to despair.

The hospital was another world entirely. Its sterile white walls stretched endlessly, interrupted only by colorful posters meant to bring cheer but somehow emphasizing the gravity of the place. The faint smell of antiseptic lingered everywhere, clinging to the air like an unwelcome guest. The waiting room was dotted with stiff chairs and quiet murmurs, a mix of anxiety and hope filling the space. The elevator ride to the oncologist's office was slow, the hum of the machinery amplifying the tension in my chest.

When I entered the doctor's office, the sight of the examination table covered in crisp white paper made my stomach churn. The cool, fluorescent lighting overhead seemed to spotlight every flaw, every ounce of fear I carried. As I sat there waiting for the doctor, I couldn't stop obsessing over the tumor. The abnormal structure of my chest had become an unwelcome focus of my life. It was impossible to hide—it jutted out just enough to be noticeable through my clothes and attempts to cover it with jewelry only aggravated the tender skin.

Out in public, I felt like every eye was on me, though I knew most people weren't paying attention. But when their gazes lingered, even for a moment, the sting of self-consciousness became unbearable. It wasn't just their glances but the questions that followed—polite inquiries that felt like daggers piercing the thin veil of my composure. "Are you okay?" "What's that?" Even well-meaning comments would send me spiraling into embarrassment. I felt like I had become a walking spectacle, my once-confident demeanor shattered by something I couldn't control.

The embarrassment didn't end with strangers. Among friends, colleagues, and even at church, I felt the weight of silent judgment. I tried to maintain a sense of normalcy, but the knot on my chest felt like a flashing neon sign, screaming for attention. Every Sunday, I wrestled with clothing choices, hoping to find something loose enough to disguise the tumor without causing discomfort. Every interaction, no matter how routine, became a minefield of insecurity. I couldn't escape the feeling that people were looking at the tumor and not at me.

Sleeping brought its own set of challenges. My favorite position—lying on my belly—was no longer an option. The pressure on the tumor caused sharp, unbearable pain, leaving me tossing and turning most nights. Turning onto my side provided only momentary relief, as even the slight friction of fabric against my chest became irritating. Sleeping on my back, though the least painful, felt unnatural and terrifying. I couldn't shake the association with the position of bodies in caskets, which only fed my growing anxiety. Nights that were once peaceful turned into long, restless battles with discomfort and fear. The lack of restful sleep began to take its toll, leaving me physically drained and emotionally fragile.

In *Invisible Battlegrounds*, Apostle Yolanda Stith highlights a crucial point: "If we don't find stability in our minds, there's no possible way we will be able to get our flesh and our spirits under control." This statement emphasizes that mental instability isn't just a psychological issue; it is deeply connected to spiritual well-being. Mental anxiety creates an environment where the body and spirit become susceptible to chaos. Without peace in our minds, our spirits struggle to align with God's will, and our flesh follows suit in disarray.

Mental anxiety is described as one of the most powerful weapons that hell wields against believers. As Apostle Stith writes, "Mental torment [dastardly spirit] is one of the biggest, if not, the biggest most powerful weapon hell routinely launches against the body of believers." Anxiety becomes a spiritual hindrance that paralyzes us emotionally, making it difficult to make wise decisions, and often leads to fear, confusion, and spiritual paralysis. The terror of the thought of death that I experienced became a tool of this torment. Anxiety wasn't just a feeling—it was a spiritual force that waged war on my peace.

The physical manifestation of my anxiety, such as vomiting at the valet or feeling an overwhelming fear at the sight of the hospital, illustrates how deeply the mind's torment can affect the body. My spirit was affected, too, as fear and anxiety clouded my faith and confidence in God's promises. This mental turmoil made it almost impossible to feel at peace or walk in faith. In the midst of this, I needed the truth of 2 Timothy 1:7 to take root in my heart: "God hath not given us the spirit of fear; but of power, and of love, and of a sound mind." This verse became my anchor, reminding me that fear is not from God, but rather, He gives us the power to overcome, the love to heal, and the soundness of mind to face any trial.

As Apostle Stith notes, "Where there is mental torment, there is the absence of peace...where there is no peace, it is almost impossible to muster up the faith to continue on your journey toward victory." Without peace, we cannot fully trust or step into God's plan for us. Anxiety not only disturbs the mind but also robs us of the spiritual peace needed to trust in God's sovereignty and purpose.

The constant disappointment opened a gate of anxiety on a level I had never experienced before. This overwhelming feeling caused me to vomit before exiting my car at the valet of the hospital. I began to taste the medicine pushed into the IV tube and almost passed out. The thick saline was clear, but the taste seemed to seep through the tube and place itself on my tongue. The atrocious smell of the alcohol pad used to clean my skin made my eyes roll to the back of my head. Although the nursing staff was incredible, the very thought of going to this excellent hospital was dreadful. Each doctor's visit chipped away at my confidence, and depression began to take hold. The repetition of bad news and the growing tumor size made me feel as though I was losing control over my own body and future. Yet, through it all, I clung to hope and faith in God's Word, even when it seemed like the only light in a very dark tunnel.

However, through God's Word and prayer, I learned to reclaim my peace. Anxiety, as a weapon of the enemy, tried to hinder my faith, but I chose to believe that my victory was already secured at the cross. Jesus' sacrifice gave me victory over fear, anxiety, and even death. I had to remind myself that no matter how terrifying the circumstances, the enemy would not win by clouding my mind with negative thoughts or medical reports.

In conclusion, mental anxiety can have a profound spiritual effect, causing emotional instability, fear, and paralysis. But by relying on God's Word, we can overcome anxiety and walk in the peace and power He has promised, knowing that our victory is already secured through Christ. The battle in the mind is real, but it is through God's peace that we gain victory in both our minds and spirits.

FAITH CONFESSION:

God sent His word (His Son, Jesus) and healed
me.

VII

I Am Healthy

To the naked eye, I looked normal; but for an entire year, the pathology report of the PET scans of my upper body stated the case of a terminally ill patient. For the first year, I expressed to the oncologist that I could perform all of my regular work and house duties with no pain. The students that accompanied the doctor looked very puzzled. Their textbook probably gave a description of how a stage three cancer patient was to look and symptoms they were to possess, but I was not their textbook character. The narrative of my condition seemed unusual, so my case was sent to the highest level within the oncology department.

Several years before being diagnosed, I wore braces, and a permanent retainer was placed on the bottom row of my teeth. On my first visit to a holistic trainer, I was asked to remove the metal retainer and any other metal I had in my body. The beginning of healing is cleaning the garbage out of the vessel: spiritually is forgiving and naturally is removing toxins out of my body. I strived every single day to stay healthy. With the holistic journey of healing, I had to change my eating habits. It was hard because my grandmother and mother are great bakers, so eliminating sugary cakes and drinks was the most difficult to remove from my diet. But I was determined to live a healthier lifestyle. I began adding more fresh vegetables to my meals and less meat. I explored different farmer's markets near my city and discovered some of the best tasting foods from the field into my basket. I began to prepare my meals in advance so that I would not be tempted to eat junk food from fast-food restaurants.

On one of my doctor's visits, the oncologist entered my examination room without a smile on his face. I began to feel sick in my stomach while trying to smile. I wanted to believe so strongly that the results of the PET scan had changed, and God had performed a miracle in my body - but that was not the case. Instead, the doctor gave me pamphlets on symptoms of chemotherapy. I continued to reject the department's treatment plan. I expected a miracle from The Most High God, but it seemed to take so long.

Against the recommendation of the oncologist, I continued to visit my local YMCA to exercise. My holistic trainer suggested that exercise would help fight off the disease and improve my strength for daily activities. I attended workout classes with senior citizens since my oncologist had recommended that I reduce any strenuous activities. To be in the same class with people 20 to 30 years older than me was embarrassing. I used smaller weights than the other chronologically mature students in my class. When attempting to follow the movements of the instructors, I noticed how weak I had become since being diagnosed. The disease growing inside of me caused me to be sluggish and forgetful, to the point that my youthfulness seemed to have been thrown out the window.

After the exercise class, I would sit in the sauna. In this hot box, I had the opportunity to share my experience with cancer with other YMCA members. So many individuals prayed with me and provided words of comfort, and some even shared their own life battles. During these moments, it seemed as if my shyness lifted off me. I was able to unfold and share my frustration with this disease, and no one abashed me when I exposed horrible descriptions of my challenges. Exercising to remain healthy was not easy. For many days, I wanted to stay home and lie on the couch to watch television, but after a while, I would see the faces of my YMCA friends on the ceiling of my condo, so I would push myself to the silver sneakers class.

Attending the YMCA and church provided a place of escape from the four walls of my condo. In church service, I was able to take the focus off of the tumor and look to the hills from where my help comes from (Psalm 121:1). Walking into the foyer to greet the saints lifted my spirit and put a huge smile on my face. The mothers and elders of the church would hug me and give me a holy kiss on the jaw. Their words of encouragement lit a fire under my feet and joy in my heart. Singing in the choir and on the praise team took me to another realm in my mind and heart. The sermons of faith and holiness confirmed my steadfast belief that God would heal me.

Many of the church members witnessed the drastic change in my body and hair, but their love and support never wavered. Throughout the entire journey, their presence was a constant source of strength. On any given week, I would receive encouraging text messages and uplifting short videos that helped keep my spirit lifted. The members of the church never ceased sharing God's word and extending their kindness to both me and my husband during this eighteen-month battle. These heartfelt gestures were more than just acts of kindness; they were a lifeline that helped keep my mind in a healthy place throughout the emotional and physical challenges of this medical ordeal.

Being from the South and coming from a large family, we did not eat the healthiest foods. For almost every area of our childhood, it was quantity over quality. We were blessed to live a short mile from my dad's mother, so during harvest times, she would get corn or collard greens from the fields of her employer. But most of the year, my mom bought vegetables in cans. We rarely ate fast food, which caused my siblings and me to be some of the best players on the PE teams. It was difficult to adjust from this way of eating, but I had to choose better food choices in order to live longer. Eating clean was not adopted by my family, which made the road to a vegetarian lifestyle much harder.

I'll never forget the day my dear friend Terri Jo visited me and asked how she could help on this health journey. As my prayer partner, I knew without a doubt that she would be lifting me up in prayer, but she wanted to do more. She told me, "I'll eat like you're eating, so you won't have to go through this health challenge alone." And that's exactly what she did. Terri bravely took on the vegetarian challenge I had embraced, walking alongside me every step of the way. Whenever we met for lunch, I could see the physical changes in her—her countenance brightened, and I noticed the weight loss as well. But it wasn't just about the food or the weight; it was about the deep, unwavering friendship and support she gave me. Terri didn't just stand by me in prayer, she truly stood with me in this battle. Her sacrifice and companionship meant the world to me. I am forever grateful for her love and the way she embraced this challenge with me, never letting me face it alone.

This change in my diet encouraged me to begin reading scriptures about the food I was eating. In Genesis 1:29, God explicitly states that He gave us "every tree, in which is the fruit of a tree yielding seed; to you it shall be for meat." While researching my condition, dietitians strongly suggested that I stop eating raw, uncooked deli meat. Preparing simple meals became a thing of the past. I had to begin cooking more vegetables and less meat. The love for cooking returned to my heart because I understood what Paul was saying in 1 Corinthians 6:19: "Know ye not that your body is the temple of the Holy Ghost?" I had to consciously put forth an effort to eat properly to honor the gift God gave me—my body. With exercise and a proper diet, I lost weight in a manner that was pleasing to my oncologist. My oncologist paid close attention to my weight to make sure it remained steady. To reduce the fear that would sneak into my mind, I would say out loud Jeremiah 30:17: "God will restore health unto me." I did all I could do to maintain my health and new lifestyle as a vegetarian. I am grateful that my family members and my best friend joined me in this massive lifestyle change.

FAITH CONFESSION:

My body is the temple of the Holy Spirit and sickness cannot stay inside of me any longer.

VIII

I Am Covered...My Hair

L isted in the chemotherapy pamphlet was the phrase: "Side effect: Hair Loss."

For 18 months, these two words—non-Hodgkin's lymphoma—terrorized me and took up too much space in my thoughts. The treatment plan my oncologist proposed came with side effects that I dreaded far more than the disease itself. Chief among them was the loss of my hair. My hair was not just strands on my head; it was tied to my sense of self, my femininity, and my spiritual identity. The thought of losing it made me reject chemotherapy, even though it could have been a crucial step in shrinking the tumor lodged under my right collarbone. At that point, the tumor didn't cause pain, but it loomed large in my mind, like the ominous antagonist in a horror story. I convinced myself that as long as my hair remained intact, I could hold onto a part of myself.

My hair journey began in childhood and was deeply rooted in tradition. From as early as I can remember, my mother would perm my sisters' and my hair, slathering the creamy substance onto our roots. We endured the burning sensation of chemical relaxers because, after the ordeal, we were rewarded with silky, straight hair—a standard of beauty we had been taught to admire. My mother had dreams of becoming a cosmetologist, but those dreams were deferred when she married and had her first child. Even though she never became a professional hairstylist, she found joy in experimenting with hairstyles on her daughters. Our hair became her canvas, and we, her willing subjects.

By the time I reached high school, my mother passed on her knowledge to us, teaching my sisters and me how to wash, style, and maintain our hair. Her teachings extended beyond technique; they carried spiritual significance. She often referenced 1 Corinthians 11:15: "But if a woman have long hair, it is a glory to her: for her hair is given her for a covering." To my mother, our hair was not just a physical attribute; it was a sacred symbol of beauty and honor. Cutting it short or straying from traditional practices felt like a betrayal of the values she instilled in us.

For years, I upheld my mother's teachings, maintaining my long, permed hair as a badge of pride. However, in my early thirties, I became curious about my natural hair texture. I wondered what lay beneath the layers of chemical treatments I had known all my life. With my husband's encouragement and a hairstylist's guidance, I made the bold decision to do the 'big chop' and cut off my permed hair to embrace my natural curls. I'll never forget the first time I looked in the mirror after the big chop. At first, I felt vulnerable—almost exposed—but as I ran my fingers through my natural curls, I saw beauty in the unfamiliar.

Over the next three years, my curls grew in abundance, and I fell in love with the versatility of my hair. Each week, I tried new styles, inspired by tutorials and tips I found online. My coworkers marveled at how I could transform my look, joking that I became a new person with each hairstyle. When I straightened my hair, it flowed longer than it ever had with perms, affirming that my hair was healthier than it had been in years. Yet, despite all the compliments and creativity, I slowly began to realize that my identity wasn't tied to my curls or length.

When cancer entered my life, it forced me to confront this truth. The thought of losing my hair initially felt like losing a part of myself. How would people see me if I no longer fit the image I had carefully curated? But through prayer, reflection, and soul-searching, I realized that I had been holding onto the wrong source of confidence. My value was not rooted in my hair, but in my spirit.

Hair is a temporary, external attribute, but the essence of who I am—my faith, my character, and my purpose—are eternal. God reminded me that "Man looks at the outward appearance, but the Lord looks at the heart" (1 Samuel 16:7). My hair didn't define me; my identity was securely rooted in Christ. Letting go of the fear of losing my hair freed me from the chains of vanity and allowed me to focus on the healing I needed—not just for my body, but for my mind and spirit.

This journey helped me understand that beauty isn't confined to societal standards, nor is it measured by what grows on my head. I am not my hair; I am a child of God, wonderfully and fearfully made. Even in the face of illness, I learned to stand confidently in this truth, knowing that my worth and identity cannot be taken away, even by cancer.

FAITH CONFESSION:

I command my hair to grow long, strong, thick
and curly!

IX

I Am Healed

After looking in the mirror for two years, the tumor was finally gone!

I AM HEALED!

Each day, I would boldly declare, "I AM HEALED!"

During the period when the tumor was growing, I couldn't wear necklaces or heavy clothing to conceal the enlarged lymph node on the right side of my chest. I also lost a significant amount of weight, and my plus-size clothes no longer fit. This led me to go on a shopping spree to update my wardrobe. Unbeknownst to me, my appetite had diminished drastically, causing me to lose weight rapidly. While I felt good and looked good, I was slowly deteriorating. Before my diagnosis, I had been intermittently working out at the YMCA near my home. Despite my efforts to exercise and adopt a healthier diet, I had struggled to lose weight. But suddenly, the pounds started to melt away. The first oncologist I saw explained to my husband and me that this sudden weight loss, without much effort, could be a sign of cancer in the body. Yet, as I gazed into the mirror, I continued to boldly affirm, "I AM HEALED."

I had to take on the mind of Christ as written in John 17:16-18, when Jesus said, "They are not of the world, even as I am not of the world. Sanctify them through thy truth: Thy Word is truth." A follower of Jesus becomes pure and holy by believing and obeying the word of God. My parents' teachings and training were to ensure that my foundation in God was solid as a rock. If God said it, I had to believe it. Regardless of the doctor's report, I believed in the word of God. The previous chapters revealed a few scriptures that I meditated on daily, which pushed me from just believing to knowing that God healed me.

There were many days when I questioned God, wondering why He was taking so long to heal my body. I even asked my oncologist if there was any way to surgically remove the enlarged lymph node. I'll never forget the day the doctor entered the examination room with the devastating news: "Mrs. Witherspoon, I've discussed your case with the heart specialist, and he advised that performing such a surgery would be too dangerous." In that moment, I felt crushed. The only medical options left were chemotherapy and radiation, and I had no choice but to face them.

During the four weeks of radiation, my lips began to darken, turning a deep, unsettling black. Despite witnessing the Word of God manifesting in my life, this physical change seemed to overshadow the progress I was making. To hide my dry, brittle lips, I started wearing dark-colored lipstick. Although it concealed the flaw, it didn't erase the embarrassment I felt. The darkness of my lips, now accentuated by the lipstick, seemed to draw attention wherever I went. It was as if everyone noticed, and many made a point of commenting on it. The frequent compliments, especially from men— "That's a pretty color on you"—only made me feel more uncomfortable and self-conscious. I remember a moment after church when the church mother, with a disapproving frown, pointed at my lips and said, "I don't like that!" Her words stung, and before I could process the hurt, she turned and walked away. Devastated, I hurried to the restroom, my heart sinking. There, I wiped away the dark lipstick, feeling a weight settle on my chest. I handed the lipstick to my mother, silently vowing never to wear dark lipstick again. That moment stayed with me for years, shaping my choices and my confidence.

Daily confessions helped to restore and maintain my reliance on God's Holy written word. My outward countenance may have shifted in a negative way, but my spirit was always lifted by the word of God. Quoting scriptures formed my thoughts about myself, my marriage, my career, and my health. According to Proverbs 18:21, "Death and life are in the power of the tongue." I stood firmly on this scripture when I said my daily confessions. When I laid in the hospital to receive treatment, I would silently say, "By His stripes I am healed" (Isaiah 53:5). When my body would break out in rashes, I would boldly declare, "God will restore me." When I felt far from God and it seemed as if my healing was farther away, I would remind God of the story of Jesus speaking healing to the Centurion man in Matthew 8:8.

During a pivotal time in my life, as I sought healing for my body and soul, I came to a profound realization about the power of God's Word. I began to understand that my struggle with cancer was not just a physical battle, but a spiritual one—a fight against generational curses that had plagued my family for decades. Through this journey, my love and steadfast belief in the Word of God grew exponentially, as I leaned on His promises and trusted in His power to break every chain.

On my father's side, I was the third generation to receive a cancer diagnosis. It seemed as though this terminal illness had woven itself into the very fabric of our family history, threatening to continue its grip on each successive generation. On my mother's side, the story was no different. I was the second generation to be diagnosed with cancer, but this time, it affected my lymph nodes, further solidifying the reality of the curse that had been passed down.

But in the midst of this struggle, I found hope and strength in the Word of God. I began to recognize that what I was facing was not just a physical ailment, but a spiritual stronghold that needed to be broken. I could not accept that this disease would define me or my family any longer. I knew that God's Word is alive and powerful, sharper than any two-edged sword, capable of piercing through the darkness and cutting off any curse that had taken root in my lineage.

I began to use Scripture as a weapon of warfare, speaking it over my life daily, declaring healing, freedom, and deliverance.

I believed that the same power that raised Christ from the dead was alive in me, and I refused to let the enemy claim victory over my body or my family's future. I stood firm on the promises of God, knowing that His Word is more than just a book—it is the living, breathing force that has the power to break every chain and set the captive free.

Through this process, I witnessed the transformation of my faith. What was once a fleeting hope became an unwavering conviction. I was no longer bound by the fear of inherited illness or the chains of my family's past. I believed that God's healing power was greater than any curse, greater than any diagnosis, and greater than anything the enemy could throw my way. I trusted that His Word would not return to Him void but would accomplish all that it was sent to do.

In the end, I found freedom. Not just from the cancer, but from the generational curse that had loomed over my family for so long. The Lord brought healing, restoration, and a new legacy—one rooted in His truth and His power to heal.

I know now that the power of God's Word can deliver anyone from any bondage, no matter how long it has been passed down. His Word is a weapon of victory, a light in the darkness, and the key to breaking every chain that would seek to hold us captive. As I continue on this journey of healing, I carry with me the knowledge that no curse is too strong, no sickness is too powerful, and no family history is beyond redemption when we stand on the promises of God's Word.

FAITH CONFESSION:

God will restore health to my body and heal me
of my wounds.

X

Disease Will Not Return

I serve the God of the Bible, whose Word and promises are true and will always come to pass. His healing power is mighty, capable of lifting those who are suffering and afflicted, restoring them to health and wholeness. God clearly expresses His desire for our well-being in 3 John 1:2, where He speaks through His servant John, saying, "Beloved, I wish above all things that thou mayest prosper and be in health, even as thy soul prospereth." This is a declaration of God's heart for us to be healthy, as it aligns with His perfect plan for our lives.

From the very beginning, God's intention was for His creation to thrive in good health. In Genesis 1:29 and Ezekiel 47:12, He provided everything we need—nutrition, life, and sustenance—so that we could walk in the fullness of His blessing and purpose. These scriptures show that God not only desires for us to prosper spiritually but also physically, in every area of our lives.

As 2 Corinthians 1:20 reminds us, "All the promises of God in Him are yea and Amen." This means that God's promises, including His promise of healing and restoration, are guaranteed in Christ. They are certain and unchangeable. Whatever He has said will be fulfilled, and His Word will accomplish what it was sent to do. I stand firmly on these truths, trusting that God's power to heal and restore is active and available for all who believe.

There were moments when doubt crept in, and the weight of fear seemed overwhelming. While I had no reason to doubt that God would do what His Word says, the reality of my situation shook me to the core. After enduring several rounds of chemotherapy and a month of daily radiation, my oncologist shared a troubling prognosis: the blood disease I had could return. He explained that, with so many lymph nodes in the body, the disease could lie dormant in other areas, undetectable by even the most advanced medical technology.

The spirit of fear tried to take hold of me, especially as I thought of my family history. Cancer had plagued my family for years, and after years of remission, I had seen it return with a vengeance in several of my relatives. I couldn't ignore the weight of that reality. The fear of recurrence was real. But I knew I had to hold on to faith, even when my heart wavered.

In that moment of doubt, I remembered the father in Mark 9:24, who, when faced with the desperation of his situation, cried out to Jesus, "Lord, I believe; help thou my unbelief." I, too, had to pray that same prayer—asking God to help me overcome the doubts and fears that threatened to paralyze my faith.

Though I was battling fear, I wasn't fighting alone. God surrounded me with a strong, loving support system— my spouse, my parents, my siblings, my prayer partners, and my church family. Together, we stood in prayer and encouragement. They reminded me of God's promises and kept me focused on His truth, not on my circumstances. With their help, I was able to push past the fear, holding tightly to the belief that God's power was greater than any diagnosis or family history.

It wasn't easy, and there were still moments when fear tried to sneak in, but I learned to trust God in the midst of my doubts. I learned that faith isn't the absence of fear, but the choice to trust God despite it. And with His help and the strength of my support team, I was able to overcome the fear and continue to walk in faith, believing that God's healing power would see me through.

God's compassion was deeply evident during my battle with lymphoma. In the most trying and uncertain moments, I could sense His loving presence guiding me, providing for me, and showing me that I was never alone. It was as if He orchestrated every step of my journey, making sure I had exactly what I needed at the right time, even in the smallest ways.

Whenever I prayed for something specific, whether it was strength, encouragement, or comfort, God would use someone from my support team to fulfill that very request. It felt as though He was personally answering my prayers through the people around me, showing His love and compassion in ways that I could never have anticipated. Whether it was a text message at just the right moment, a prayer spoken over me, or a word of encouragement, I saw the hand of God moving in my life daily.

Psalm 91:14 says, "Because he hath set his love upon me, therefore will I deliver him: I will set him on high, because he hath known my name." This verse became a powerful declaration over my life during my fight with lymphoma. God's love for me, His compassion, was the foundation of my hope and strength. He didn't leave me in my distress; He promised deliverance and protection because I had set my heart upon Him. His love and care were not just abstract concepts but real, active forces in my life, working for my good.

Daily, I confessed Nahum 1:9, which says, "What do ye imagine against the Lord? He will make an utter end: affliction shall not rise up the second time." This verse became a powerful weapon in my battle against fear. The fear of the lymphoma returning was very real, but as I spoke this promise over my life, I felt the weight of fear begin to crumble. God had promised that affliction would not rise again, and I stood firm on that promise, rejecting the fear and replacing it with faith in His Word.

Being adopted as a child of God gave me the confidence to claim these promises, knowing that what God had spoken over the children of Israel was just as much for me. I wasn't a stranger or outsider to His love and care—I was His child, and He had made me a part of His covenant promises. This identity as His child encouraged me to boldly apply His promises to my own life, trusting that just as He had delivered others, He would deliver me.

God's compassion wasn't just a feeling—it was action. He showed me His love through the people He placed around me, through the promises He spoke to my heart, and through His daily provision and peace. Through it all, I knew that He cared deeply for me and would bring me through this trial, not only to heal my body but to strengthen my spirit and deepen my trust in Him. His compassion is limitless, and His promises are sure. I stand today, healed and whole, a testimony of His unwavering love and faithfulness.

Giving honor to God has firmly established my confidence, not just in ministry, but in every aspect of my life—my career, my industry, and beyond. I know that when I honor God, He opens doors and grants me favor, positioning me among great men and women who share His calling and purpose. As the Apostle Paul beautifully expresses in 2 Corinthians 4:17 (KJV), "For our light affliction, which is but for a moment, worketh for us a far more exceeding and eternal weight of glory." This reminds me that no matter what trials or afflictions I face, they are temporary, and they cannot compare to the eternal rewards and glory God has for me.

My confidence in God's Word is a shield against the doubts and fears that the symptoms of the disease might bring. I refuse to let them dictate my life or control my future. I know that God's promises are greater than any sickness or disorder. While Satan may try to cripple me with fear, pain, or disease, I stand on the truth that God's rewards, His blessings, and His healing are far more powerful and enduring.

Isaiah 58:11 is a verse that continues to strengthen me: "And the LORD shall guide thee continually, and satisfy thy soul in drought, and make fat thy bones: and thou shalt be like a watered garden, and like a spring of water, whose waters fail not." This verse reassures me that, no matter the circumstances, God will guide me, sustain me, and refresh me. His provision is continual, His satisfaction is complete, and His healing is everlasting. Like a well-watered garden, I will flourish, nourished by His Word and His presence, because His promise is that His waters will never fail.

In all of this, my confidence is rooted in the unshakeable truth of God's Word. I am not defined by illness or affliction but by the eternal and abundant life He has promised to those who trust in Him. The power of daily confessions of healing scriptures was transformative in my journey. With every word I spoke, life began to enter what had once been a place of sickness and despair. The Word of God is alive, and as I declared His promises over my life, it breathed life into my body, particularly into my blood, which had been ravaged by illness. These confessions were not mere words—they were declarations of faith that carried the power to shift the atmosphere around me and within me.

Every time I spoke healing scriptures, I felt the power of God's Word catapult me into a new revelation of healing, where I saw beyond the physical symptoms and embraced the truth of God's promise for restoration. I began to understand that the Word of God is not just something we read; it is something we activate and speak into our circumstances. As I confessed His Word daily, I was reminded of His authority over sickness and disease, and I believed that His healing power was at work within me.

The act of confessing healing scriptures daily was like planting seeds of faith, and over time, those seeds took root and produced the fruit of healing. I saw God's Word shift my perspective, transform my mind, and empower my spirit to rise above the affliction. His Word has the ability to resurrect what is broken, restore what is lost, and bring new life where there was once death. Through my daily confessions, I experienced this truth firsthand, and it became clear to me that God's Word has the power to heal, to restore, and to set us free.

FAITH CONFESSION:

The Lord God, Jehovah Rapha, has healed me of lymphoma and this disease will not return to my body according to Nahum 1:9. In Jesus Name!

References

Bible, KJV

Invisible Battlegrounds, Yolanda Stith

The Intercessor's Dictionary Words & Phrases,
Terri Jo Davis

https://truevinepublishing.org/the-intercessors-dictionary

Anatomy & Physiology by Lindsay M. Biga, Sierra Dawson, Amy Harwell, Robin Hopkins, Joel Kaufmann, Mike LeMaster, Philip Matern, Katie Morrison-Graham, Devon Quick & Jon Runyeon is licensed under a Creative Commons Attribution-ShareAlike 4.0 International License, except where otherwise noted.